Keto Meal Prep

Contents

INTRODUCTION 8

CHAPTER 1: WHAT IS KETO ALL ABOUT? 9

CHAPTER 2: STRATEGY AROUND MEAL PREP 15

CHAPTER 3: GET INSPIRED! MEAL PREP IDEAS. 18

CHAPTER 4: MISTAKES THAT YOU CAN AVOID 20

CHAPTER 5: 7 OF THE MOST ASKED QUESTIONS ABOUT MEAL PREPPING. 21

CHAPTER 6: YUMMY BREAKFAST RECIPES .. 23

Cheesy Egg and Bacon Cups 23

Delicious Ham and Cheese Waffles 24

Cinnamon and Coconut Porridge 26

Supreme Baked Eggs and Avocado 28

A Very Berry Smoothie 29

The Original Denver Omelette 30

Fancy Deviled Eggs 32

Nutritious Smoothie for The Morning 33

Easy Mushroom Frittata 34

CHAPTER 7: LIKE SEAFOOD? YOU WILL LOVE THESE RECIPES 37

Grilled Shrimp and Avocado 37

Brie Packed Smoked Salmon 38

Ecstatic Garlic and Butter Cod 40

Mediterranean Tuna Salad 41

Dark and Broody Tilapia 42

Cucumber and Avocado Salmon Bites 44

Sassy Broccoli Tilapia 46

Sensibly Smoked Salmon with Dill Spread 48
    Tomato Stuffed Tuna Balls 49

CHAPTER 8: SNACKS RECIPES...........................50

Herb Dressed Chicken Parmesan Fingers...........................50

Bacon Moza Sticks 52

The fantastic Buffalo Chicken Dip..53

Amazing Chipotle Kale Chips...55

Simple Fine Granola..56

Raspberry and Cheesy Pops 57

Awesome Buffalo Drumsticks 58

Tuna Croquettes 60

Deep Walnut Bites 61

CHAPTER 9: POULTRY RECIPEE IDEAS. 62

Unbelievably Healthy Chicken Lettuce Wraps 62

Chicken & Cabbage Platter..64

Heavenly Turkey Balls...65

Grilled Chicken and Mozzarella Spinach 67

Skinny Turkey Wrap..68

Balsamic Chicken and Vegetables 70

Salsa Chicken Bites 71

Turkey, Grape and Pecan Salad 72

Buffalo Chicken Lettuce Wraps 74

CHAPTER 10: RED MEAT RECIPEES 76

Cheesy Avocado Steak Patties 76

Bacon Burger Bombs 77

Bacon Stuffed Jalapeno 78

Asian Beef Steak 80

Mexican Beef Zucchini Boats 82

Steak and Broccoli Medley 84

Caramel and Pork"Rind" Cereal 85

Pepper and Sausage Soup 86

Generous Skirt Steak and Cilantro Lime 87

CHAPTER 11: VEGETARION RECIPES 89

Hungry Turtle's Caesar Salad 89

Satisfying Spinach Dip 90

Satisfying Ginger Soup 91

Personal Veggie Pizza 92

Fancy Charred Garlic Artichokes 94

Healthy Cauliflower Curry 95

Great Sautéed Zucchini 97

Fancy Charred Garlic Artichokes 98

Cool Cucumber Soup 100

Extremely Healthy Guacamole 101

Crunchy Cauliflower Rice 102

CHAPTER 12: DESERT MY FAVORITE 105

Pumpkin and Cardamom Donuts 105

Blueberry Morning Scones 106

Deliciously Chocolate Coated Bacon 108

Easy Bake Coconut Macaroons 109

Secret Yogurt Parfait 112

Creamy and Satisfying Vanilla Pudding 114

CONCLUSION 116

Introduction

There's a really famous saying that goes something like this"Failing to Prepare is Preparing is Fail" Straightforward words which hold a deep significance! Despite the fact that it can sound a little harsh at first, when you look at it carefully and try to enjoy the deeper feeling, then you'd observe that this line is something of a universal truth! Proper preparing can allow you to win half the battle! And the value of the concept goes up ten folds when contemplating cooking! Especially in an age where we are all going through a super hectic schedule with no time to cook healthy meals! If you're among these, then this is the book for you! The core aim of the publication is to not only offer you a plethora of unique recipes to follow but also work as a one-stop guide that you completely understand the concepts of both the Ketogenic Diet and Meal Prepping. Bearing this in mind, I've dedicated the first few chapters to present the fundamental concepts of Ketogenic Diet and Meal Prepping, which can be followed by the 71 easy to comprehend recipes, all to help you grasp your stove and make very own masterpiece. I hope that you like this book and find the recipes offered in this publication helpful and delicious!

Chapter 1: What Is Keto All About?

Understanding Ketogenic Diet During your day to day life, you've definitely heard of the word "Ketogenic" where there appears to occur a discussion about healthy diets! Because you're already reading this book, I presume that you're also one of those people that are interested in getting to know more about this astonishingly adequate diet that's changing the lives of thousands worldwide! So, let us begin with the most fundamentals. What's Ketogenic Diet To completely understand the fundamental theories of Ketogenic Diet, you must first understand a little bit about the term "Keto" itself. The term "Keto" is derived from a natural metabolic process called "Ketosis," which forms the heart of the Ketogenic Diet. To further understand the functioning procedure which goes behind the Ketogenic Diet, you must first learn how to appreciate the fact that if our body is exposed to a substantial amount of Carbohydrate, it gradually starts to raise the quantity of Glucose and Insulin and discharge them in our blood. It's a really well-known actuality that Glucose is the most readily convertible molecule that's present in our body and is therefore used for energy by default. The insulin on the other helps to keep the Glucose in our blood. Well, Here is the thing. Whenever sugar is present in abundance in your body, it also drastically reduces the quantity of fat that's burned through hard work because the body consistently favors to break down glucose rather than fat to get their energy. This is also one reason why you may not be getting satisfactory results even after hours upon hours of workout sessions! However, as you reduce your Carbohydrate intake, it gradually enters into a stage called"Ketosis" that is basically the body's natural reaction mechanism which allows it to handle low food intake. In this phase, a considerable number of ketones are generated that causes the body to burn more fat rather than Carbohydrate whenever the body needs energy. So, when you begin to deprive your body of carbs, the body starts to automatically find other resources it may use to acquire the required energy. Since fat is present in abundance in our body, it instantly turns its focus to burning fat. Whenever carbohydrates aren't easily available, the liver begins t break down fat into fatty acids, which can be further broken down into energy-rich substances called"Ketones." This entire process is called Ketosis! A deeper look into Ketones When your body decides that it's time to start burning fat, the body takes the fat into the liver where it's broken down into glycerol and fatty acids via a process called Beta-Oxidation. Given enough time, the body gradually begins to fully adapt itself to utilize these ketones as a source of energy, and the muscles learn how to convert the acetoacetate to Beta-Hydroxybutyrate (BHB for short), that's the body's preferred Ketogenic supply of energy to the brain. Asides from this, acetone can also be generated, which the body expels as waste. The glycerol generated during the beta-oxidation goes through a process called gluconeogenesis that converts the glycerol into glucose which the body uses for energy. Alternatively, the extra protein obtained through a Keto diet can also be used for energy by converting them. This permits the body to fulfill the minimum need of Glucose of your system without even using carbohydrates to receive it! The way to know you're in Ketosis if you're a newcomer, then it may be hard for you to tell if your body has entered into a state of Ketosis or not. These are rules of thumb that will assist you detect if your body is in Ketosis. Your mouth will feel dry, and you feel have increased thirst the amount of washroom visits increases as you may need to urinate more frequently. Your breath will have a slight"Fruity" odor that will resemble that of a nail polish Apart from these three, you'll find the feeling mentioned previously of having a minimal hunger level and increased physical energy. Maintaining optimal ketosis levels. Now naturally it's possible to reduce down your carbohydrate intake and input Ketosis! However, some specific guidelines will permit you to input Ketosis in no time and allow you to keep it for a protracted period. Maintain your daily carbohydrate intake under 20 carbohydrates Keep your protein levels at around 70g per day Do not starve! Swallow adequate degree of fat. Bear in mind that the body will need fat to burn fat. Stay away from snack times and stick with your breakfast, lunch and dinner dishes with nothing in between. That being said, below are the benefits you will enjoy while adhering to a suitable Ketogenic Diet! Not Go For Attempt to avoid dried fruits that are high in sugar content Drinks Go For Water Black Coffee Unsweetened and Herbal Teas Nut Milks Light Beet Wine Not Go For Drinks like Pepsi or Coke High Fructose Syrup Nectar Honey Sodas Sweets Go For Stevia Xylitol Erythritol Inulin Monk Fruit Powder Cocoa Dark

Chocolate The significant benefits of Ketogenic Diet A proper Keto diet can enable you to lower the amount of bad cholesterol so to stop arterial blocks from happening Energy taken from burning off body fat will keep you lively because body fat is present in abundance in our body the degree of LDL will decrease which will make the body less likely to suffer with Type-2 Diabetes You won't always feel hungry Ketosis helps improve skin condition and protect against skin or acne inflammation from happening. But apart from that, you're apparently interested in realizing the connection the between the way the Keto Diet promotes weight loss right? Here is how: A Ketogenic Diet significantly increases the caloric consumption of the body that ultimately contributes to weight loss promotion whenever you're limiting the quantity of carbohydrate ingestion of your body, you're also restricting yourself from different food and finally lower the calorie intake as well that a crucial component for weight loss. Through the practice of Gluconeogenesis, as mentioned earlier, the body begins to burn even more carbohydrates protein and fat into carbohydrates to support the body by providing it with sufficient energy. The procedure itself will also help burn additional calories each and every day. Ketogenic Diet promotes the creation of Appetite suppressant hormones like Leptin and ghrelin which functions to decrease the sensation of hunger, enabling you to go through the day by eating less food. A Ketogenic diet directly helps to improve the amount of fat burnt throughout the entire day through exercise and daily activities But there are some unwanted effects you ought to know about as well. During this period, there's a possibility that you might experience some minor distress. You don't need to get alarmed though as these will finally pass away within a couple weeks. Mental fogginess Headaches Keto-Flu Aggravation Dizziness Ketosis causes the body to drop a substantial amount of electrolytes, which can be one of the prime causes of the above-mentioned symptoms. Asides from those however, you will find specific side effects you might face as well! Same as before, no need to be alerted as they will pass away finally within the first fourteen days, after your body habituates itself into the diet. Symptoms may include: Frequent urge to urinate Hypoglycemia Constipation Increased Sugar Craving Diarrhea Sleep problem hints and mistakes to avoid Now you're almost ready to start off your trip! But below are a couple of quick tips which can allow you to Kickstart your Keto diet pursuit effortlessly. Purchase a counter to keep track of your carbohydrate intake. Toss out all the high-carb creates from your kitchen. Pack up your pantry with just Keto suitable produces. Makeup and stick to a strict meal plan Attempt to give your old customs and pursue newer, healthier habits. Keep yourself packaged up with sufficient water to be certain you could replenish the flushed-out electrolytes. As soon as you've decided that you will jump right into a Ketogenic Diet, 1 thing that you may find interesting to follow along is a technique called"Occasional fasting" This lets you know that you ought to begin a pre-phase of low carbohydrate diets before really starting the diet , to allow your body to adjust and re-orient itself to the forthcoming changes. This fasting technique is comprised of two stages.

Namely the Construction Stage (Time between first and last meal) and the cleaning period (Time between first and last meal). Attempt to keep 12 hours between the cleanup phase and 8 hours between the construction phases to begin with. Then continue growing from that. Easy steps may include ✓ Drinking organic broth if possible ✓ Taking a just a pinch of pink salt with you consumed foods ✓ Adding about 1/4 teaspoon of pink salt to 16 oz of water consumed ✓ Adding vegetables such as kelp into your dishes ✓ Eating up vegetables like celery or cucumber for a more natural way to sodium replenishment It's essential to keep a proper exercise regimen to ensure that your body is at tip-top shape throughout the regime. With everything said and done, it ought to be mentioned today that there are a number of common mistakes that are produced by new Keto fans. We often get confused concerning the simple fact of how many carbs they can eat daily. The very necessary standard carb count is that you ought to keep your carbohydrate intake somewhere around 20-50g with a maximum intake of 100-150g at best. Too much protein will cause the body to begin burning up protein rather than Fat! So, try to maintain a balance. A grave mistake that people makes is they sometimes attempt to reduce the Fat intake also, thinking it will double the effectiveness of a Ketogenic Diet. However, that's entirely incorrect, and you shouldn't skip out on your fat consumption. Be certain that you go for as much water as possible. As you're on a Ketogenic Diet, the body will begin to flush away electrolytes that will make you weak. To tackle this impact, it is vital to keep your body hydrated constantly and have a ideal quantity of salt also.

Chapter 2: Strategy Around Meal Prep

Meal Prep Basics In the simplest terms, Meal Prepping is the method of producing a strategic blueprint or"Layout" of those foods that you're likely to follow during a week that's compatible with the diet that you're following. In even simpler terms, Meal Prepping is the process of planning what you will eat and how can you create that, beforehand to spare more time and money. The core objective and benefits of Meal Prepping are as follows: This can enable you to save a bucket load of money by letting you make a rough estimate of your cost ahead of time that it enables you to stick to a healthy meal plan, the Ketogenic Meal Plan such as! Meal Prepping helps reduce food wastage It will help to clear off your mind by eliminating the strain of"What to cook next" since everything is intended of time If you keep mixing up your weekly plans with unique meals, it is going to allow you to prevent monotony Meal Prepping will enable you to control your portions by adjusting a set amount of food per mealthis is going to give you greater control of your diet and promote weight loss Greater control of your food routine can allow you to make a more balanced and nutritious diet program in the future Since everything is pre-planned, it is going to enable you to avoid the rush of "Last minute preparations" and make the cooking process more comfortable for you Meal Prepping will enable you to multitask with other important functions, rather than sitting at the kitchen all day to cook. Because you will keep everything ready, it is going to save a whole lot of time from your everyday routine and let you concentrate on other activities. Must have kitchen essentials Below are a few of the vital equipment that you may want to keep handy. Cutting Boards: Attempt to have boards which are made from solid materials such as glass, plastic, rubber or marble! These are largely rust resistant, and the non-porous surface makes it easier to wash them than wood. Tools and Equipment: the simplest ones include Measuring cups: Needed to measure out spices and condiments. Variously sized spoons: The multiple sized strands will permit you to measure out small quantities of spices. Glass bowls and non-metallic containers: They're necessary for storing the meat . Packaging materials (mentioned previously): The substances are cited above, and they can be used to keep the meat in the refrigerator. Cold Storage Space (the refrigerator will suffice): Since the meats need to be kept under 40 degrees Fahrenheit, a refrigerator should be sufficient. Always be certain that you use a sharp knife hold a knife under your arm or put it under a piece of meat Always keep your knives within visible distance Always keep your knife down point Always cut towards the very surface and away from the body Never allow children to toy with knives unattended Wash the knives while cutting different kinds of food Mesh glove for security: Cutting the meat demands precision as you'll use a very sharp knife. The following kinds of the glove should be kept in mind: Rubber gloves Butchering Gloves Mesh Glove Kitchen Scale for dimension: A kitchen scale will permit you to get precise measurements of marginally pieces of meat and condiments. Internal Thermometer: A meat thermometer can enable you to assess the internal temperature of the jerky to make certain you could guarantee that the jerky is prepared. Baking Sheet: These are flat, rectangular metal pan that's used in an oven, chiefly for flat goods like sheet cakes, biscuits, etc.. Colander: A colander is a bowl-shaped kitchen utensil with pockets which permits you to drain food like pasta or rice. These are also utilised to rinsed veggies. Aluminum Foil: Also called misnomer tin foil, these are utilized to wrap up and cover meals. But while going out to buy containers, you might notice there are usually two different types of containers, plastic, and glass. For Glass Glass containers are somewhat more expensive but are best for long-term storage on account of their heavy weight, glass containers aren't perfect for"on-the-go" ingestion They are easier to clean If you're worried about plastic security, then these are the ones to go with! For Plastic Easy to carry and lightweight, perfect for people that are constantly on the go They're more convenience and come in a huge selection of sizes and shapes they're simple to dispose Asides from plastic and glass, you can also see that there are Steel containers. Steel containers are excellent if you would like to keep foods in the freezer since they help to prevent freezer burn.

Chapter 3: Get Inspired! Meal Prep Ideas.

Amazing Meal Prep Ideas bear in mind that Meal Prep ideas aren't set in stone! The following are only a few of the countless different Meal Prep ideas which you're can get all around the net! The principal goal of them is to inspire you and provide you a base of Meal Preps! Make a plant beforehand: If you're reading this publication, then you've probably decided to go on a sterile Eating diet journey. A fantastic way to start off this is to begin with a few of recipes, for maybe 7 days. Choose which recipes you're going to use and create a rough thought inside your mind. Make a list and purchase the ingredients accordingly beforehand. But also, for keeping healthy salads! Assuming that you're a nutritious buff, it may be a great idea to prepare your salads beforehand and keep them in mason jars. Be sure that you keep the salad dressing in the bottom of the jar to make certain that nothing greens do not get soggy! Three-way seasoning in 1 pan: If your diet plan needs you to stay with lean meats like chicken, then seasoning them from time to time might become somewhat of a chore. A simple solution to this would be to prepare a pan with aluminum foil dividers. Using these will let you season three or more (depending on the number of dividers you're using) forms of chicken seasoning to be achieved using the exact same pan! Boil eggs in an oven rather than a pot: Now this may sound a bit odd at first, but it's highly effective! The issue here comes with the amount of eggs which may be boiled in 1 go. If you're using a standard sized pot, then you'd most likely have the ability to squeeze in 5 or 6 eggs maximum in 1 batch. However, if you attempt to bake your eggs in muffin tins with an oven, then you might have the ability to have a dozen or perfectly hard-boiled eggs very quickly! Keep your ready smoothies suspended in muffin tins: Plopping out a number of ingredients early in the morning may be a chore for some people. This will not just save time but will also provide you with a great dose of satisfaction as you awake in the morning and throw a few "smoothie cups" to the blender for a simple yet wholesome breakfast. Roast vegetables that require exactly the same time in 1 batch: When you're preparing large batches of vegetables for roasting, it's intelligent to go ahead and produce batches of vegetables based on how long they take to roast. Learn to efficiently use a skewer: When you think of skewers, you automatically consider kabobs! But Skewers are not necessarily intended to be used only with road meats. Wooden skewers can allow you to quantify how much meat you're going to consume in 1 go. Thus, you can punch in your meat in numerous skewers and divide them equally and keep them for the remainder of the week. These can effortlessly give you enough room to separate each and every part of your meal while making certain you don't mix up everything and make a mess. The different ingredients would also be simple to find and use! Keep a tab of your achievements: This might be the vital component of a Meal Prepping routine. Always be certain that you measure your progress and set little milestones that you accomplish. Alternatively, taking a look at your positive progress will greatly inspire you to push ahead as well Now you have a basic grasp of the concepts of Ketogenic Diet and Meal Prepping let me give you a breakdown of only some of the awesome advantages of Meal Prep!

Chapter 4: Mistakes that you can avoid

Mistakes to Avoid and A Note on Weight Loss irrespective of how experienced we are, as human beings, we're bound to make mistakes more frequently than not! Don't keep your meals for too long out as they may easily get infected with germs of germs, Do not rush when washing and washing your veggies. Take your time and thoroughly clean your veggies before processing them. You should always be certain that you're heating your meals properly. Overheating them will burn them up while not heating them will leave damaging bacteria on the surface of the food. Here is the thing, the potency of Meal Prepping about weight loss largely depends upon the sort of diet that you're after, which in our case is a Ketogenic Diet! However, the subsequent meal prepping strategies can enable you to improve the outcome of the total diet that you're following. Always try to keep your veggies chopped up in advance and keep them in separate containers. Try to create and prepare foods which can be kept in your refrigerator for later use. Prepare the snacks that you're going to eat for the rest of the week and then inventory them up. Snacks are great when it comes to curbing the appetite with only a single bite. Rather than boiling or cooking your vegetables, try to roast them in massive batches over the weekend. It can allow you to preserve their nourishment and will encourage you to consume them generously since they would be easily available, which would also greatly be contributing to cutting your calories down. Try to stay healthy condiments around the home like olive oil, salsa, soy sauce, lemon, flavored vinegar and so on... Remember that these are merely to give you an idea of the flexibility of a proper Meal Plan. You aren't restricted to only these! Keep on exploring and produce your Meal Plan strategies that will complement the diet that you're following.

Chapter 5: 7 Of the Most asked Questions about meal prepping.

Meal Prep Tips and FAQs With all that said, the next section covers some of the most often asked questions! If this is the first time, then it is almost certain you are going to have some questions concerning Meal Prep. Allow me to clear some of the most frequent ones for you before allowing you to enter the recipes! Q1. How long can food usually last? As a guideline, 4-5 times is an outstanding period to maintain your meals healthy in airtight containers stored in refrigerators. Nonetheless, you might refer to the link below for additional information.
https://www.fda.gov/downloads/food/foodborneillness contaminants/ucm109315.pdf Q2. How should you store dinner prepped food? Plastic/Glass/Steel containers are great to keep cooked food. Just be certain that you allow your foods cool for 30-40 minutes prior to moving to your container and sealing them. Q3. A buffet meal prep is when you pile cook a few different ingredients and create meals throughout the week as you continue going, rather than prepping all the meals simultaneously. Q4. Q5. How should you inspire yourself to meal prep each week? You should bear in mind that Meal Prep can help you save a whole lot of time while letting you follow a healthful diet (in our case, Ketogenic Diet) and maintain a healthy body! And of course, it is going to allow you to save a bucket load

of cash also! Q6. While freezing meals aren't recommended (as re-heating them sometimes reduces the taste), you're more than welcome to chill sauces, soups, chilis, etc. and thaw them when required. Q7. How can you re-heat workweek lunches without destroying them? While in the office, use your workplace Microwave to warm up your food. And that pretty much covers the fundamentals of Meal Prep! With that said, you're now ready to explore the recipes!

Chapter 6: Yummy Breakfast Recipes
Cheesy Egg and Bacon Cups
Serving: 6
Prep Time: 10 minutes
Cook Time: 15 minutes
- Ingredients 6 bacon strips
- 6 large eggs
- A handful of fresh spinach
- 1/4 cup cheese
- Salt and pepper to taste

How To
1. Pre-heat your oven to 400-degree Fahrenheit
2. Fry bacon in a skillet over moderate heat, drain the oil and keep them on the side
3. Take muffin tin and grease with oil
4. Line with a slice of bacon, press down the bacon well, making certain the ends are sticking out (to be utilized as handles)
5. Take a bowl and beat eggs
6. Drain and pat on the spinach dry
7. Add the spinach to the eggs
8. Insert a quarter of the mixture at all your muffin tins
9. Sprinkle cheese and season Bake for 15 minutes
10. Enjoy!

Possible to stay in the box for 3-4 days.
- Fat 7 grams
- Net Carbohydrates: 1 grams
- Protein: 8 Grams
- Calories 102

Delicious Ham and Cheese Waffles

Serving: 2
 Prep Time: 10 minutes
Cook Time: 4 minutes per waffle
Ingredients
- 8 whole eggs
- 1 tsp baking powder
- Basil and paprika to taste
- 2 oz cheddar cheese, grated
- 2 oz ham steak, chopped
- 1 tsp salt
- 12 tbsp of melted butter

How To
1. Take two bowls and decode 4 eggs separating the white and simmer, keep the remaining side
2. Add salt, butter, baking powder into the egg yolk, whisk well
3. Gradually fold to the yolk
4. Whisk egg whites well and season with salt, keep whisking until stiff
5. Fold half of the egg whites into egg yolk and let it sit for several minutes Fold in remaining egg whites
6. Add a little the batter into your waffle maker and cook for 4 minutes each waffle
7. Repeat with the remaining batter
8. when the batter is completed, make more using the remaining eggs if preferred Enjoy!

Nutrition (Per Serving)
Calories: 620
Fat: 50g

Net Carbohydrates: 1g
Protein: 45g

Cinnamon and Coconut Porridge

Serving: 4
Prep Time: 5 min
Cook Time: 5 minutes
Ingredients
- 2 cups of water
- 1 cup of 36-percent heavy cream
- 1/2 a cup of unsweetened dried coconut, shredded
- 2 tbsp of oat bran
- 2 tbsp of flaxseed meal
- 1 tablespoon of butter
- 1 plus a 1/2 teaspoon of stevia
- 1 teaspoon of cinnamon
- Sea salt as needed
- Toppings such as blueberries or banana slices

How To
1. bring the above-mentioned ingredients into a small pot, mix well until completely integrated
2. Transfer the pot to your stove over medium-low heat and bring the mixture to a slow boil
3. Stir well and remove the heat
4. Divide the mixture into equal portions and let them sit for 10 minutes
5. Top with your desired toppings and enjoy!

Nutrition (Per Serving)
Calories: 171

Fat: 16g
Net Carbohydrates: 6g
Protein: 2g
Storage Options/Meal Prep Tips: Though these are best served hot, it's still possible to keep them for up to two days in mason jars. Be sure that you keep them in your fridge.

Supreme Baked Eggs and Avocado

Serving 4
Prep Time: 10 minutes
Cook Time: 15
Ingredients

- 4 whole eggs
- 2 avocado, sliced halved lengthwise and stoned
- A pinch of garlic powder
- A pinch of salt
- A pinch of pepper
- a bit of parmesan cheese, grated

How To

1. Pre-heat your Oven to 350-degree Fahrenheit
2. Cut avocado and scoop a quarter of the flesh
3. Add into muffin tin
4. Season the avocado halves
5. Break the egg and squirt to each half of the avocado and sprinkle cheese
6. Place the avocado in oven and bake for 15 minutes
7. Take them and out of the oven serve with a scatter of the scooped out avocado flesh.

Nutrition (Per Serving)
Calories: 158
Fat: 16g
Net Carbohydrates: 1g
Protein: 3g
Storage Options/Meal Prep Tips: Cover with aluminum foil to store them in your refrigerator for up to two days.

A Very Berry Smoothie

Serving: 1
Prep Time: 4 minutes
Cook Time: 0 minutes
Ingredients
- 1/4 cup of frozen blueberries
- 1/4 cup of frozen blackberries
- 1 cup of unsweetened almond milk
- 1 teaspoon of vanilla bean extract
- 3 teaspoon of flaxseed
- 1 spoonful of chilled Greek yogurt
- Stevia as needed

How To
1. Mix everything in a blender and emulsify them
2. Pulse the mixture four time till you have your preferred thickness
3. Pour the mix into a glass and enjoy!

Nutrition (Per Serving)
Calories: 221
Fat: 9g
Net Carbohydrates: 8g

Protein: 21g

Storage Options/Meal Prep Tips: Its best to serve the smoothie refreshing, however it is still possible to prepare the ingredients ahead. Add milk and vanilla extract and mix them in 1 cup containers and keep them in your refrigerator. In terms of the berries, store them in freezer bags. The flaxseed and stevia can be combined and stored in zip bags also.

The Original Denver Omelette

Serving: 1
Prep Time: 4 minutes
Cook Time: 1 minute
Ingredients
- 2 tbsp of butter
- 1/4 cup of sliced onion
- 1/4 cup of green bell pepper,
- diced 1/4 cup of halved grape tomatoes
- 2 whole eggs
- 1/4 cup of sliced ham

How To
1. Take a small skillet and set it over medium heat
2. Add butter and allow the butter to melt
3. Add onion and bell pepper and Saute for three or four minutes
4. Take a bowl and whip eggs
5. Insert the remaining ingredients and stir
6. Add sautéed onion and peppers and stir
7. Microwave the egg mix for 1 minute

8. Serve and enjoy!

Nutrition (Per Serving) Calories: 605

Fat: 46g

Net Carbohydrates: 6g

Protein: 39g

Storage Options/Meal Prep Tips: You can pre-cook the onion and pepper and keep them in zip bags before the morning that you would like to make the omelet. Same is true for the chopped ham, store zip bags and put in your fridge.

Fancy Deviled Eggs

Serving: 2

Prep Time: 9 minutes

Cook Time: 11 minutes

Ingredients

- 4 whole hard boiled eggs
- 2 tbsp of mayonnaise (Keto friendly or homemade)
- 1 tbsp of spicy brown mustard
- 1 tablespoon of diced green chilies

How To

1. Boil your eggs for 9 minutes
2. Transfer boiled eggs into a water bath and peel skin
3. slice the egg in half and scoop out the yolks
4. Take a bowl and add yolks, mayonnaise, chilies and mustard
5. Mix well and transfer the mixture back to the egg white cubes
6. Enjoy!

You may store the boiled eggs in airtight containers for seven days in your refrigerator and use when required.

Nutritious Smoothie for The Morning

Serving: 3
Prep Time: 10 minutes
Cook Time: 0 minutes
Ingredients
- 1/2 of a avocado, pitted and peeled
- 7 oz of total fat unsweetened coconut milk
- 1 cup of baby kale, chopped
- 1/2 a cup of lemon, diced
- 2 tbsp of freshly squeezed lemon juice
- 2 tbsp of freshly squeezed orange juice
- Water as needed

How To
1. bring the above-mentioned ingredients into a blender
2. Blend on low until everything is mixed well
3. Boost to high and mix until smooth
4. Add several drops of liquid stevia for extra taste
5. Divide the mixture into 3 servings and enjoy!

Can be stored in airtight containers for up to 3 days.

Easy Mushroom Frittata

Serving: 6
Prep Time: 9 minutes
Cook Time: 44 minutes
Ingredients
- 2 tbsp of butter
- 12 whole eggs
- 4 oz baby spinach, diced

- 3/4 cup of fontina cheese, diced
- 1/2 a cup of red onion, chopped
- 1 cup mushrooms, sliced
- 1/2 a cup Greek yogurt, plain
- 1/8 tsp of nutmeg

How To
1. Pre-heat your oven to 350-degree Fahrenheit
2. Take a iron skillet and set it over medium heat
3. Add butter and allow the butter melt
4. Add mushrooms and onion and cook till translucent
5. Take a bowl and whip eggs, sour cream and spinach
6. Add /12 a cup of cheese
7. Add butter to the skillet with mushroom and onion and set it over medium
8. Pour egg mixture and let it cook for 4 minutes (no stir fry)
9. Eliminate heat and sprinkle remainder of the cheese
10. Transfer to oven and bake for 29 minutes
11. Serve and enjoy!

Nutrition (Per Serving)
Calories: 359
Fat: 14g
Net Carbohydrates: 14g
Protein: 43g
Storage Options/Meal Prep Tips: Transfer to airtight containers and serve when necessary, potential to store for seven days.

Chapter 7: Like Seafood? You Will Love These Recipes

Grilled Shrimp and Avocado

Serving: 6
Prep Time: 20 minutes
Cook Time: 5 minutes
Ingredients
- 2 whole avocados, pitted, peeled and cubed
- 2 pound of shrimp, peeled and deveined
- 1/2 a cup of berries, chopped
- 1/2 a cup of bell pepper, chopped
- 1/2 a cup of onion, chopped
- 4 tbsp of olive oil
- 2 tsp of freshly squeezed lime juice
- 1 teaspoon of garlic powder
- 1 teaspoon of sea salt
- 1/4 tsp of fresh ground black peppper

How To
1. Place your grill to medium-high heat
2. Take a bowl and add garlic powder, half of salt and pepper and olive oil
3. Mix well
4. Add shrimp to the bowl and chuck
5. Take a salad bowl and add bell pepper, tomato, onion, avocado and lime juice with salt and toss
6. Cook the shrimp on your grill for 3 minutes each side
7. Divide the mixture and salad and enjoy!

Nutrition (Per Serving)

Calories: 409
Fat: 25g
Net Carbohydrates: 11g
Protein: 36g
Storage Options/Meal Prep Tips: Cover the portions and store in your refrigerator for up to 3 days. Be certain that you re-heat before serving ! If you freeze this you can get 4-6 months.

Brie Packed Smoked Salmon

Serving: 4
Prep Time: 4 minutes
Cook Time: 0 minutes
Ingredients
- 8 oz Brie round
- 1 tbsp of fresh dill
- 2 tbsp of lemon juice
- 4 oz Smoked Salmon

How To
1. Slice Brie in half length wise
2. Spread salmon, dill and lemon juice over the Brie
3. Place the other half on top
4. Serve with Celery sticks/ cauliflower bites
5. Enjoy!

Nutrition (Per Serving)
Calories: 241
Fat: 19g Net
Carbohydrates: 0g

Protein: 18g

Storage Options/Meal Prep Tips: Transfer to airtight containers and serve when necessary, potential to refridgerate for 3-4 days.

Ecstatic Garlic and Butter Cod

Serving: 3
Prep Time: 5 min
Cook Time: 20 minutes
Ingredients
- 3 cod fillets, 8 oz each
- 3/4 pound of baby bok choy, halved
- 1/3 cup of thinly sliced butter 1 plus a 1/2 tbsp of minced garlic
- Sea salt as needed
- Freshly ground black pepper

How To
1. Pre-heat your toaster to 400-degree Fahrenheit
2. Cut 3 sheet of aluminum foil, large enough to accommodate 1 fillet
3. Place cod fillet on each of the sheet and add garlic and butter on top of the fillets
4. Add bok choy and season with salt and pepper according to your taste
5. Fold the package and garnish them in pouches Organize in your baking sheet Bake for 20 minutes and then transfer to cooling rack

Be certain that you re-heat in oven before serving. Freezer 4-6 months.

Mediterranean Tuna Salad

Serving: 6
Prep Time: 15 minutes
Cook Time: 0 minutes
Ingredients
- 10 oz of endives, leaves split
- 15 oz of solid white albacore tuna packed in oil, drained
- 1 plus a 1/2 cups of feta cheese, crumbled
- 3/4 cup of extra virgin olive oil
- 3/4 cup of diced roasted red pepper
- 1/3 cup of quartered green olives
- 1/3 cup of fresh parsley, choppped
- 1 plus a 1/2 tbsp of freshly squeeze lemon juice
- 1 plus a 1/2 tbsp of drained capers
- Red pepper flakes as needed
- Fine sea salt as needed
- Fresh ground black pepper, as needed

How To
1. Take a bowl and add tuna, crumble
2. Fold into feta cheese, roasted red pepper, green olives, lemon juice, parsley, capers, olive oil and combine
3. Season with salt and pepper
4. Add red pepper flakes for spiciness
5. Enjoy!

Nutrition (Per Serving)
Calories: 352
Fat: 26g
Carbohydrates: 5g
Protein: 25g

Storage Options/Meal Prep Tips: For keeping, divide the mixture into six pieces in air tight containers and include endive leaves on top to cover them. Refrigerate for up to 3 days and serve chilled when required.

Dark and Broody Tilapia

Serving: 2
Prep Time: 9 minutes
Cook Time: 9 minutes
Ingredients
- 1 cup of cauliflower, chopped
- 1 teaspoon of red pepper flakes
- 1 tablespoon of Italian seasoning
- 1 tablespoon of garlic, minced
- 6 oz of tilapia
- 1 cup of English cucumber, chopped with peel
- 2 tbsp of olive oil
- 1 sprig dil, sliced
- 1 teaspoon of stevia
- 3 tbsp of lime juice
- 2 tbsp of Cajun blackened seasoning

How To
1. Take a bowl and add the seasoning ingredients (except Cajun)
2. Add a tbsp of oil and whip
3. Pour dressing over celery and cauliflower
4. Brush the fish with olive oil on both sides
5. Take a skillet and grease it well with 1 tbsp of olive oil
6. Press Cajun seasoning on both sides of fish

7. Cook fish for 3 minutes each side
8. Serve with veggies and enjoy!

Nutrition (Per Serving)
Calories: 530
Fat: 33g Net
Carbohydrates: 4g
Protein: 32g

Storage Options/Meal Prep Tips: Keep the cooked fish in 1 zip tote along with the veggies and dressing in a different, great for 3-4 days. Serve when needed by blasting everything and microwaving for 30 minutes. Freezer time 4-6 months.

Cucumber and Avocado Salmon Bites

Serving: 5
Prep Time: 15 minutes
Cook Time: 0 minutes

Ingredients
- 1 large cucumber, sliced into 10 bits of 1/3 inch rounds
- 1 large whole avocado
- 8 oz of cream cheese
- 4 oz of cooked red slamon, flaked
- 1 tablespoon of freshly squeeze lemon juice
- 1/2 a tbsp ofchopped green onion
- Tabasco sauce

How To
1. Halve the avocado carefully and take out the stone
2. Scoop out the flesh and then transfer to a bowl

3. Add cream cheese and mash the avocado nicely
4. Add lemon juice and mix
5. Season with Tabasco sauce
6. Arrange cucumber slices on platter and divide the avocado cream cheese mixture on top
7. Split the flaked red between bits and garnish with green onion.

Sassy Broccoli Tilapia

Serving: 1
Prep Time: 4 minutes
Cook Time: 14 minutes
Ingredients
- 6 oz of tilapia, frozen
- 1 tablespoon of butter
- 1 tablespoon of garlic, minced
- 1 teaspoon of lemon pepper seasoning
- 1 cup of broccoli florets, fresh

How To
1. Pre-heat your oven to 350-degree
2. Insert fish in aluminum foil packets
3. Arrange lettuce about fish
4. Sprinkle lemon pepper on top
5. Close the loaf and seal
6. Bake for 14 minutes
7. Take a bowl and add butter and garlic, mix well and keep the mix on the side
8. Remove the packet from oven and transfer to platter Place butter on top of the broccoli and fish, serve and enjoy!

Nutrition (Per Serving)
Calories: 362
Fat: 25g
Net Carbohydrates: 2g
Protein: 29g
Storage Options/Meal Prep Tips: You may prep the ingredients ahead by add garlic and butter into a small zip bags along with the cut broccoli in a different zip tote. In terms of the lemon pepper, keep them in a little container. Freezer 4-6 months.

Sensibly Smoked Salmon with Dill Spread

Serving: 8
Prep Time: 20 minutes
Cook Time: 0 minutes
Ingredients
- 4 oz of smoked salmon
- 4 oz of full fat cream cheese, room temperature
- 2 and a 1/2 tablespoon of mayonnaise (Keto Friendly or Homemade)
- 2 tbsp of chopped fresh dill
- Sea salt as needed
- Freshly ground black pepper
- Cucumber and tomatoe wedges for serving

How To
1. Add smoked salmon, cream cheese, mayonnaise into a food processor and pulse
2. Pour mixture into airtight container and mix in fresh dill

3. Season accordingly and function with cucumber/tomato wedges
4. Enjoy! Serve with carrot, celery or cucumber sticks.

Freezer 2-3 months.

Tomato Stuffed Tuna Balls

Serving: 2
Prep Time: 25 minutes
Cook Time: 0 minutes
Ingredients
- 8 tomatoes, medium
- 1 tablespoon of capers
- 2 -- 3 oz cans of tuna, drained
- 10 Kalamata olives, pitted and minced
- 2 tbsp of parsley
- 1 tbsp of olive oil
- 1/2 a teaspoon of thyme
- Salt and pepper as needed

How To
1. Line a cookie pan with paper towel and scoop guts from the Tomatoes
2. Maintain the tomato cubes on the side
3. Take a bowl and combine olives, thyme, parsley, pepper in a bowl and mix
4. Add oil and blend
5. Fill out the tomato shells with carrot mixture

Chapter 8: Snacks Recipes

Herb Dressed Chicken Parmesan Fingers

Serving: 6
Prep Time: 15 minutes
Cook Time: 30 minutes
Ingredients
- 2 pounds of boneless and skinless chicken breast
- 4 garlic cloves, peeled and sliced
- 4 oz of butter
- 1 cup of freshly grated parmesane cheese
- 2 tbsp of chopped fresh coriander
- 1 teaspoon of chili pepper flakes
- Sea salt as needed
- Freshly ground black pepper

How To
1. Pre-heat your Oven to 350-degree Fahrenheit
2. Coat a baking sheet with non-stick cooking spray
3. Take a saucepan and set it over medium-heat
4. Add butter and melt the butter, swirl to coat well
5. Stir in garlic and Sauté until fragrant, remove the heat and maintain the garlic on the side for 15 minutes
6. Take a bowl and add rosemary, chili pepper, parmesan cheese, pepper and stir well

7. Rinse the chicken breast thoroughly and blot it dry with kitchen towel
8. Slice into 24 finger shaped pieces and coat in the butter and garlic mix
9. Dredge the pieces from the cheese mix and organize them in your baking sheet
10. Bake for 25-30 minutes until the fingers are golden brown
11. Transfer them to a cooling rack and let them cool

Nutrition (Per Serving)
Calories: 370
Fat: 20g
Net Carbohydrates: 6g
Protein: 40g
Storage Options/Meal Prep Tips: Move the Chicken Fingers to an airtight container and refrigerate for up to two days. Freezer safe for 2-6 months.

Bacon Moza Sticks

Serving: 4
Prep Time: 10 minutes
Cook Time: 5 minutes
Ingredients
- 8 bacon strips
- 4 mozarella string cheese bits
- Suflower oil, as needed

How To
1. Take a heavy-duty skillet over moderate heat and add about 2 inches of oil

2. Heat it up into 350-degree Fahrenheit
3. Have each string cheese to 8 bits
4. Wrap each piece of string cheese with strip of bacon and fasten using toothpick
5. Cook the sticks in oil for 2 minutes until the bacon is browned
6. Put the sticks on plate lined with kitchen towel and drain
7. Serve!

Nutrition (Per Serving)
Calories: 278
Fat: 15g
Net Carbohydrates: 3g
Protein: 32g
Storage Options/Meal Prep Tips: Transfer to airtight containers and serve when necessary, potential to refrigerate for 3 days. Freezer 3-4 months.

The fantastic Buffalo Chicken Dip

Serving: 4
Prep Time: 19 minutes
Cook Time: 9 minutes
Ingredients
- 6 whole eggs
- Water
- 6 oz chicken, cooked
- 3 tbsp of maynnaise (Keto Friendly/ Homemade)
- 1 and a 1/2 tbsp of red buffalo wing sauce (sugarfree)

- 1/4 cup of blue cheese, crumbled
- 8 celery stalks

How To
1. Boil eggs for 9 minutes and let them cool
2. Peel and dice the eggs
3. Chop the cooked chicken finely
4. Slice celery to 2-inch-long pieces
5. Take a bowl and add all the ingredients except celery
6. Mix well
7. Blend the celery sticks with the mix and serve with more hot sauce

Nutrition (Per Serving)
Calories: 286
Fat: 20g
Net Carbohydrates: 2g
Protein: 19g
Storage Options/Meal Prep Tips: Transfer the filling to airtight containers and serve when necessary, potential to refrigerate for 3-4 days. Maintain celery in zip bags.
Nutrition (Per Serving)
Calories: 235 Fat: 17g
Net Carbohydrates: 6g
Protein: 8g
Storage Options/Meal Prep Tips: Transfer to airtight zip bags and serve when necessary, potential to refrigerate for 3-4 days.

Amazing Chipotle Kale Chips

Serving: 4
Prep Time: 4 minutes

Cook Time: 29 minutes
Ingredients
- 2 large bunch kale, chopped into 4 inch pieces and stemmed
- 1 tbsp of olive oil
- 1/8 tsp of salt
- 1 teaspoon of chipotle powder
- 1/4 cup of parmesan cheese, shrdded

How To
1. Wash the kale thoroughly and dry them, cut into 4-inch pieces
2. Pre-heat your oven to 250-degree Fahrenheit
3. Take 3 baking sheets and line the with parchment paper
4. Take a bowl and add kale, coat with olive oil, cheese and chipotle
5. Put on baking sheet
6. Bake for 19 minutes and then assess crispiness
7. Bake for 9 minutes longer if needed
8. Enjoy!

Nutrition (Per Serving)
Calories: 37
Fat: 3g
Net Carbohydrates: 3g
Protein: 1g Storage
Options/Meal Prep Tips: Transfer to airtight containers and serve when necessary, potential to refrigerate for seven days.

Simple Fine Granola

Serving: 4

Prep Time: 16 minutes
Cook Time: 0 minutes
Ingredients
- 1 oz cocao Sacha Inchi Seeds
- 1 oz gureyere cheese, finely chopped
- 1 oz pepitas, roasted

How To
1. Take a zip bag and include all the listed ingredients
2. Mix well and serve
3. Enjoy!

Nutrition (Per Serving)
Calories: 449
Fat: 34g
Net Carbohydrates: 3g
Protein: 25g
Storage Options/Meal Prep Tips: Transfer to airtight containers and serve when necessary, potential to refrigerate for seven days.

Raspberry and Cheesy Pops

Serving: 8
Prep Time: 20 minutes
Cook Time: 0 minutes
Ingredients
- 1/4 cup of cream cheese
- 1/4 cup of sliced fresh raspberries
- 4 tbsp of coconut oil
- 4 tablespoon of heavy cream
- 4 tbsp of butter

- 1 teaspoon of pure vanilla extract

How To
1. Add cream cheese, coconut oil, butter in a bowl
2. Mix well and microwave in 10 seconds interval until the cheese has melted
3. Remove the bowl and stir it.
4. Stir in heavy cream and fold in chopped raspberries
5. Stir in vanilla additional into the mixture and stir
6. Pour the mixture into ice cube tray for 16 segments Chill for two hours and serve!

Awesome Buffalo Drumsticks

Serving: 4
Prep Time: 10 minutes
Cook Time: 40 minutes
Ingredients
- 2 pound of chicken wings
- 2 tablespoon of olive oil
- 2 tbsp of white wine vinegar
- 1 tbsp of tomato paste
- 1 teaspoon of salt
- 1 teaspoon of paprika powder
- 1 tbsp of tabasco

For Chili Aioli
- 2/3 cup of mayonnaise
- 1 tbsp of smoked paprika
- 1 garlic clove, minced

How To
1. Pre-heat your oven to 450-degree Fahrenheit

2. Put drumstick in plastic bag
3. Mix the other ingredients in a small bowl and pour the marinade into the plastic bag
4. Shake the bag well and enable the chicken to marinate for 10 minutes
5. Take a baking dish and coat it with oil Transfer drumstick to baking dish and bake for 30-40 minutes
6. Take another bowl and combine aioli ingredients, serve with drumstick!
7. If you would like, then you add some carrot and cucumber sticks too!

Refrigerate for 2-3 days. Do not store the aioli mix, make the mix before serving. Freezer 2-6 months Satisfying

Tuna Croquettes

Serving: 4
Prep Time: 4 minutes
Cook Time: 9 minutes
Ingredients
- 1 can of tuna, drained
- 1 whole large egg
- 8 tbsp of grated parmesan cheese
- 2 tbsp of flax meal
- Dash of salt
- Dash of pepper
- 1 tbsp of minced onion

How To
1. bring all the ingredients into a blender (except flax meal) and pulse them mix to a crispy texture

2. Form patties with the mix
3. Dip both sides of the patties in flax meals and fry them in hot oil until both sides are browned well

Nutrition (Per Serving)
Calories: 105
Fat: 5g
Net Carbohydrates: 2g
Protein: 14g
Storage Options/Meal Prep Tips: Store the patties in airtight containers and keep in refrigerator for 2-3 days. Freezer 2-3 months.

Deep Walnut Bites

Serving: 10
Prep Time: 10 minutes
Cook Time: 2 minutes
Ingredients
- 6 oz of freshly grated Parmesan cheese
- 2 tbsp of chopped walnuts
- 1 tbsp of unsalted butter
- 1/2 a tbsp of chopped fresh coriander

How To
1. Pre-heat your oven to 350-degree Fahrenheit
2. Take two large rimmed baking sheets and line with baking paper
3. Add parmesan cheese, butter into a food processor and combine
4. Add walnuts into the mix and pulse Take a tablespoon and scoop mix onto the baking sheet

5. Top with chopped coriander
6. Bake for eight minutes and then transfer to cooling rack Allow it to cool for 30 minutes Serve and enjoy!

Nutrition (Per Serving)
Calories: 80
Fat: 3g
Net Carbohydrates: 7g
Protein: 7g
Storage Options/Meal Prep Tips: Store in airtight container and serve when necessary, refrigerate for up to 5 Days. Freezer 2-3 months.

Chapter 9: Poultry Recipee Ideas.

Unbelievably Healthy Chicken Lettuce Wraps

Serving: 10
Prep Time: 10 minutes
Cook Time: 2 minutes
Ingredients
- Chicken breast, diced into 1 inch pieces
- A cup of mushrooms, diced
- Half a cup of water chestnuts diced
- 1 tbsp of Olive oil
- 1 tbsp of teriyaki Sauce
- A dash of garlic powder
- A dash of onion powder
- A dash of pepper
- A dash of cayenne pepper
- Salt as needed Pepper as needed
- Tomato and cucumber slices for ganrish

How To
1. Take a skillet and put it over Medium heat
2. Add all the listed Ingredients (except lettuce) and cook for 10 minutes until the chicken is Cooked thoroughly
3. Transfer the mixture to a Platter and shred the chicken Move The mix to lettuce leaves and roll
4. Insert few slices of tomatoes and cucumbers

Nutrition (Per Storage Options/Meal Prep Tips:

After cooking, store the components in Zip bag or airtight containers and keep in refrigerator. Serve by wrap in lettuce leaves.

Chicken & Cabbage Platter

Serving: 10
Prep Time: 10 minutes
Cook Time: 2 minutes
Ingredients
- Half a cup of Onion, sliced
- 2 tbsp of Sesame garlic Flavored oil
- 4 cups of shredded Bok-Choy
- 1 cup of fresh bean sprouts
- 3 stalks of cleery, chopped
- 1 plus a 1/2 teaspoon of minced garlic
- 1 teaspoon of stevia
- 1 cup of chicken broth
- 2 tbsp of coconut aminos
- 1 tbsp of freshly minced ginger
- 1 teaspoon of arrowroot
- 4 boneless chicken breast, cooked and chopped Thinly

How To
1. Shred the cabbage
2. Slice Onion and place on Platter alongside rotisserie chicken
3. Insert A dollop of mayonnaise on top and drizzle olive oil over the cabbage
4. Season with salt and pepper according to a taste
5. Enjoy!

Store in airtight containers for 1 week and function as needed by microwaving for A couple of minutes

Heavenly Turkey Balls

Serving: 2
Prep Time: 10 minutes
Cook Time: 27 minutes
Ingredients
- 2 Pound ground turkey
- One ounce of ork rind
- 3 little red Spinach
- 3 sprigs of thyme
- 2 large whole eggs
- 1 oz pork rinds
- Half of a medium green pepper
- One smallish onoin
- Half a teaspoon of salt.
- Half a teaspoon of pepper
- Two cups of spinach
- Ten slices of bacon.

How To
1. Take a baking sheet protect it with a Foil and toss on your bacon
2. Pre-heat Your oven to a temperature of 400-degree Fahrenheit
3. Once fully warmed, toss in the bacon on your Oven and cook for 30 minutes until finely crisped

4. While the bacon has been cooked, take all of The other ingredients and throw them in a food processor and dice them as Required
5. Toss in all the ingredients Except the bacon on top of the ground turkey mix and finely blend them
6. After the bacon is done, take it out and drain The fat
7. Form about two - meatballs and lay Them over precisely the identical sheet of bacon
8. Finely Cook up the meatballs for 20 minutes before the juice run clear
9. Skewer about 2-3 pieces of bacon around each
10. And combine the bacon fat, spinach, seasoning of your choice and produce of Stick to function as a side with your meatball.

15g Protein: 25g Storage Options/Meal Prep Tips: Move to Air tight containers and shop for 3-4 days.

Grilled Chicken and Mozzarella Spinach

Serving: 6
Prep Time: 5 min
Cook Time: 10 Minutes
Ingredients
- 3 large chicken breast, sliced half lenghtwise
- 10 ounce spinach, frozen and drained
- 3 oz mozzarella cheese, part skim
- 1/2 a cup of roasted red peppers, cut in long Strips

- 1 teaspoon of olive oil
- 2 garlic cloves, minced
- Salt and pepper as needed

How To
1. Pre-heat your Oven to 400-degree
2. Slice chicken breast Lengthwise
3. Take a skillet and And cook spinach and garlic in oil for 3 minutes
4. Put chicken on the skillet pan and top with spinach, roasted peppers and cheese
5. Bake until the cheese melts.

Nutrition (Per Serving)
Calories: 195 Grams
Fat: Seven Grams
Net Carbohydrates: Three Grams
Protein: thirty grams
potential to refrigerate for 4 days.

Skinny Turkey Wrap

Serving: 6
Prep Time: 10
minutes Cook Time: 10 minutes
Ingredients
- 1 plus a 1/4 Onions, minced
- 1 tbsp of olive oil
- 1 garlic clove, minced

- 2 tsp of chili paste
- 8 oz water chestnut, diced
- 3 tbsp of hoisin sauce
- 2 tbsp of coconut aminos
- 1 tablespoon of rice vinegar
- 12 butter lettuce leaves
- 1/8 tsp of salt

How To
1. Take a pan and put it over medium Heat
2. Add garlic and turkey into the Pan
3. Heat for 6 minutes before the turkey Is cooked well
4. have a bowl and add In hoisin sauce, coconut aminos, vinegar and chili paste
5. Transfer the mixture and divide between lettuce Leaves
6. Serve and enjoy!

Nutrition (Per Serving)
Calories: 162
Fat: 4g
Net Carbohydrates: 7g
Protein: 23g

Storage Options/Meal Prep Tips: Store in airtight containers and refrigerate for up to 5-7 days before served! Be sure that you keep mix and lettuce leaves in separate containers.

Balsamic Chicken and Vegetables

Serving: 4
Prep Time: 15 minutes
Cook Time: 25 minutes

Ingredients
- 8 chicken thigh, boneless and skinless
- 10 stalks of asparagus, halved
- 2 peppers, cut in chunks
- 1 red onion, diced
- 1/2 a cup of carrots, sliced
- 2 garlic cloves, minced
- 5 oz mushrooms, diced
- 1/4 cup of balsamic vinegar
- 2 tbsp of olive oil
- 1/2 a teaspoon of stevia
- 1/2 tablespoon of oregano
- Salt and pepper as needed

How To
1. Pre-heat your toaster to 425-degree Fahrenheit
2. Take a bowl and add all of The veggies and mix
3. Add spices and Oil and blend
4. Dip the chicken pieces into Spice mix and coat them well
5. Set the Veggies and chicken on a pan in one layer
6. Cook for 25 minutes Serve and enjoy!

Nutrition (Per Serving)
Calories: 401
Fat: 17g
Net Carbohydrates: 11g
Protein: 48g

Salsa Chicken Bites

Serving: 1

Prep Time: 4 minutes
Cook Time: 14 minutes
Ingredients
- 2 chicken breast
- 1 Cup salsa
- 1 taco seasoning mix
- 1 cup plain Greek Yogurt
- 1/2 a cup of cheddar cheese, cubed

How To
1. Take a skillet and put it over medium heat
2. Add chicken breast, 1/2 cup of salsa and taco seasoning
3. Mix well and Cook for 12-15 minutes until the chicken are done
4. Take out the chicken breast and dice them Put the pieces on toothpick and top with Cheddar
5. Put yogurt and remaining salsa In cups and use as dips Enjoy!

Nutrition (Per Serving)
Calories: 359
Fat: 14g
Net Carbohydrates: 14g
Protein: 43g

Turkey, Grape and Pecan Salad

Serving: 4
Prep Time: 10 minutes
Cook Time: 15 minutes
Ingredients
- 1 plus a 1/2 pounds turkey, ground

- 2/3 cup mayonnaise (Keto-Friendly/ Homemade)
- 2/3 cup pecans, chopped
- 1 cup red grapes, halved
- 6 celery stalks, diced
- 1/2 a teaspoon of salt
- 1/2 a teaspoon of pepper

How To
1. Cook the turkey in a pan and allow it brown
2. Take a bowl and add grapes, celery bits and pecans
3. Season with salt and Pepper
4. Add mayonnaise and blend
5. allow the turkey cool and slice it
6. Add turkey slices to the salad mix and toss Enjoy!

Nutrition(Per Serving)
Calories: 150
Fat: 20g
Net Carbohydrates: 6g
Protein: 8g
Storage Options/Meal Prep Tips: Transfer to airtight containers and serve when needed, potential to refrigerate for 5 days.

Buffalo Chicken Lettuce Wraps

Serving: 2
Prep Time: 35 minutes
Cook Time: 10 minutes

Ingredients
- 3 chicken breast, boneless and cubed
- 20 pieces of butter lettuce leaves
- 3/4 cup cherry tomatoes, halved
- 1 avocado, chopped
- 1/4 cup green onions, diced
- 1/2 a cup of ranch dressing
- 3/4 cup hot sauce

How To
1. Take a mixing bowl and add chicken Cubes and hot sauce, blend
2. Place in refrigerator And allow it to marinate for half an hour
3. Pre-heat your toaster to 400-degree Fahrenheit
4. Place coated chicken on cookie pan and bake For 9 minutes
5. Build lettuce serving cups with equal amounts of lettuce, green onions, tomatoes, ranch dressing and cubed chicken Serve and enjoy!

Nutrition (Per Serving)
Calories: 106
Fat: 6g
Net Carbohydrates: 2g
Protein: 5g
Storage Options/Meal Prep Tips: Transfer to airtight containers and serve when needed, potential to refrigerate for 5 days. Maintain the lettuce and other components alongside Chicken in separate containers to prevent sogginess.

Chapter 10: Red Meat Recipees

Cheesy Avocado Steak Patties

Serving: 2
Prep Time: 15 minutes
Cook Time: 10 minutes
Ingredients
- 1 lb of 85% lean ground beef
- 1 small avocado, pitted and peeled
- 2 pieces of yellow cheddar cheese
- Salt as needed
- Fresh ground black pepper as needed

How To
1. Pre-heat and prepare your broiler to high
2. Divide beef into 2 equal sized patties
3. Season the patties with salt and pepper
4. Broil the patties for 5 minutes each side Transfer the patties to a platter and add cheese Slice avocado into pieces and put them on top of the patties enjoy!

Nutrition (Per Serving)

Calories: 568

Fat: 43g

Net Carbohydrates: 9g

 Protein: 38g

Storage Options/Meal Prep Tips: Once cooked, you can save them by wrapping the patties in aluminum foil and keeping them on your fridge, good for 3-4 days. Be certain that you re-heat them before serving with strips of avocado. Freezer 3-4 months.

Bacon Burger Bombs

Serving: 4
Prep Time: 10 minutes
Cook Time: 60 minutes
Ingredients
12 slices of bacon
12 cubes of 1-inch sized smoked cheddar cheese
12 rounds of 1-ounce raw sausage patties
Salt as needed
Cumin as needed
Onion powder as needed
Pepper as needed
How To

1. Pre-heat your oven to a temperature 350-degree Fahrenheit
2. Lay your sausage rounds on a cookie sheet lined up with parchment paper
3. Dust the sausages with onion powder, cumin, salt and pepper
4. Insert pieces of cheese in the center portion of your rounds
5. Form a ball all over the cheese with sausage and then roll them up together, giving them a solid shape
6. Wrap the bacon around your sausage chunks
7. Bake for approximately 60 minutes in 350-degree Fahrenheit Have fun eating!

Nutrition (Per Serving)
Calories: 312
Fat: 16g
Net Carbohydrates: 18g

Protein: 11g

Storage Options/Meal Prep Tips: Transfer to airtight containers and serve when necessary, potential to simmer for 5 days.

Bacon Stuffed Jalapeno

Serving: 2
Prep Time: 15 minutes
Cook Time: 10 minutes
Ingredients
- 12 large jalapeno peppers
- 16 bacon strips
- 6 oz of full fat cream cheese
- 2 tsp of garlic powder
- 1 teaspoon of chili powder

How To
1. Pre-heat your oven to 350-degree Fahrenheit
2. Place a wire rack over a roasting pan and keep it to the side
3. Create a sliced lengthways across jalapeno pepper and scrape out the seeds, then discard them
4. Put a nonstick skillet over high heat and add half your bacon strip, then cook until crispy
5. Drain them
6. Chop the cooked bacon strips and transfer to large bowl
7. Add cream cheese and mix
8. Season the cream cheese and bacon mix with garlic and chili powder

9. Mix well
10. Materials the mixture into the jalapeno peppers together and wrap raw bacon strip all around
11. Arrange the stuffed wrapped jalapeno on prepare cable rack
12. simmer for 10 minutes
13. Transfer to cooling rack and enjoy!

Nutrition (Per Serving)
Calories: 209
Fat: 9g
Net Carbohydrates: 15g
Protein: 9g
Storage Options/Meal Prep Tips: Transfer to airtight containers and serve when necessary, potential to refrigerate for 5 days.

Asian Beef Steak

Serving: 2
Prep Time: 4 minutes
Cook Time: 4 minutes
Ingredients
- 2 tbsp of sriracha sauce
- 1 tbsp of garlic, minced
- 1 tbsp of ginger, freshly grated
- 1 yellow bell pepper, cut in strips
- 1 red bell pepper cut in thin strips
- 1 tbsp of sesame oil, garlic flavored
- 1 tbsp of stevia
- 1/2 a teaspoon of curry powder

- 1/2 a teaspoon of rice wine vinegar
- 8 oz of beef sirloin cut into pieces
- 2 cups of baby spinach, stemmed
- 1/2 head of butter of lettuce, torn

How To
1. Add garlic, sriracha sauce, 1 tsp of sesame oil, rice wine vinegar and stevia bowl
2. Mix well
3. Pour half of this mixture into zip bag and include beef, let it marinade
4. Assemble the brightly colored salad by coating the vegetables in 2 bowls in the following sequence: baby spinach, butter lettuce, two peppers on top
5. Remove the beef from marinade and discard the liquid
6. Heat up sesame oil in skillet over moderate heat and add beef, stir fry for 3 minutes
7. Transfer your stove beef in addition to the salad
8. Drizzle another half of your curry mixture Sprinkle sriracha sauce on top and serve!

Nutrition (Per Serving)
Calories: 350
Fat: 23g
Net Carbohydrates: 4g
Protein: 28g

Storage Options/Meal Prep Tips: It's possible to store the steak and salad individual in zip bags in your refrigerator and function by assembling them. Be certain that you not exceed 2-3 days of refrigeration time. Freezer 3-4 months.

Mexican Beef Zucchini Boats

Serving: 4
Prep Time: 5 min
Cook Time: 20 minutes

- Ingredients 1 pound of ground beef
- 2 tbsp of olive oil
- 1 teaspoon of salt
- 2 tbsp of Tex-Mex seasoning
- 1 teaspoon of salt
- 1/2 a cup of finely chopped fresh cilantro
- 1 tbsp of olive oil
- 2 zucchini
- 1 and 1/4 cups of shredded cheese

How To

1. Pre-heat your toaster to 400-degree Fahrenheit
2. Split the zucchini in half-lengthwise and eliminate the seed
3. Season with salt and let them sit for 10 minutes
4. Take a frying pan and set it over medium heat
5. Add olive oil and allow the oil heat up
6. Add ground meat and season with salt and Tex-Mex seasoning
7. Cook until the liquid has evaporated
8. Blot off drops of liquid with kitchen towel
9. Put zucchini halves in a greased baking dish
10. Mix 1/3rd of the cheese into ground beef alongside finely chopped cilantro, mix well
11. Divide the mixture between your Zucchini ships

12. Sprinkle cheese on top
13. Bake for 20 minutes
14. Let them cool for 5 minutes Enjoy!

Steak and Broccoli Medley

Serving: 4
Prep Time: 5 min
Cook Time: 15 minutes
Ingredients

- 4 oz of butter
- 3/4 pound of ribeye steak
- 9 oz of broccoli
- 1 yellow nion
- 1 tbsp of coconut amions
- 1 tablespoon of pumpkin seeds
- Salt as needed
- Pepper as needed

How To
1. Slice the beef and onions
2. Chop broccoli (including the stem)
3. Take a frying pan and put it over medium heat, add butter and permit the butter to melt
4. Insert meat and season with salt and pepper according to your taste
5. Maintain the meat on the side
6. Add walnut broccoli and onion to the same pan and add more butter Add coconut aminos and move the meat back Stir and season with Serve with a dollop of butter and pumpkin seeds

Freezer time 3-4 months.

Caramel and Pork"Rind" Cereal

Serving: 4
Prep Time: 40 minutes
Cook Time: 10 minutes
Ingredients
- 1 oz Pork Rinds
- 1 cup unsweetened vanilla coconut mik
- 2 tbsp of butter 2 tablespoon of heavy cream
- 1 tbsp Eryhtrytol
- 1/4 tsp of cinnamon, ground

How To
1. Take a pan and put it over medium heat
2. Add 2 tbsp of butter and allow the butter melt
3. Eliminate heat and add Erythritol
4. Set heat to moderate and keep stirring until the caramel mixture starts to bubble
5. Fold in pork rinds and stir
6. Transfer entire mix to container and cover with foil, freeze for a while
7. Serve with milk and a spoonful of nuts
8. Serve and enjoy!

Pepper and Sausage Soup

Serving: 2
Prep Time: 10 minutes
Cook Time: 45 minutes
Ingredients
- 32 ounce Pork sausages
- 1 tbsp olive oil

- 10 ounce raw spinach
- 1 medium Green Bell Pepper
- 1 can jalapenos with tomaotes
- 4 cup beef stock
- 1 tbsp of chili powder
- 1 tbsp of cumin
- 1 teaspoon of garlic powder
- 1 teaspoon of italian seaosning
- 3/4 tsp of salt

How To
1. Take a large sized pot and set it over medium heat
2. Add olive oil and allow the oil to warm up
3. Add sausages and cook until seared all around
4. Slice the green pepper into small pieces and add to the pot
5. Season with salt and pepper
6. Add tomatoes and jalapenos and stir
7. Add spinach on top and cover with lid, then wait until the spinach has wilted
8. Insert the rest of the spice and broth
9. Let it cook for thirty minutes over medium-low heat
10. Remove the lid and simmer for 15 minutes Serve and enjoy!

Nutrition (Per Serving)
Calories: 525
Fat: 4g Net
Carbohydrates: 2g
Protein: 27g

Storage Options/Meal Prep Tips: Store the portions in airtight containers for about 2-3 days.

Generous Skirt Steak and Cilantro Lime

Serving: 3
Prep Time: 45 minutes
Cook Time: 10 minutes
Ingredients
- 1 pound of Skirt Steak
- 1/4 cup of coconut aminos
- 1/4 cup of Olive Oil
- 1 medium sized lime, juiced
- 1 teaspoon of garlic, minced
- 1 small sized Handful Cilantro
- 1/4 tsp of Red Pepper Flakes For the Cilantro Paste
- 1 teaspoon of garlic, minced
- 1/2 a teaspoon of Salt
- 1 cup of gently refreshing cilantro
- 1/4 cup of olive oil
- 1/2 a medium sized lemon, juiced
- 1 medium sized deseeded Jalapeno
- 1/2 a teaspoon of Cumin
- 1/2 a teaspoon of Coriander

How To
1. Remove the outer silver skin off the skirt steak
2. Take a plastic bag and add the Cilantro Lime Steak marinade ingredients into the bag, add the beef and mix to coat it up
3. Permit it to simmer for 45 minutes in your refrigerator

4. Make the sauce by adding the paste ingredients into a food processor and pulse until blended to a paste Take a iron skillet and put it over medium-high heat
5. Remove the beef from the bag transfer beef into the pan and sear both sides (each side for 2-3 minutes)
6. Serve with the skillet sauce on top Enjoy!

Nutrition (Per Serving)
Calories: 432
Fat: 32g
Web Carbohydrates: 4g
Protein: 38g

Chapter 11: Vegetarion Recipes

Hungry Turtle's Caesar Salad
Serving: 6
Prep Time: 15 minutes
Cook Time: 0 minutes
Ingredients
- 12 cups of rommain lettuce, chopped
- 1/3 cup of extra virgin olive oil
- 1/3 cup of fresh grated parmesan cheese
- 3 tbsp of freshly squeezed lemon juice
- 1 plus a 1/2 tablespoon of mayonnaise (Keto-Friendly/Homemade)
- 1/3 tsp of garlic powder freshly ground black pepper

How To

1. Take an Air Tight container and add lemon juice, garlic powder, olive oil, mayonnaise and combine
2. Split the mixture in 6 servings
3. Take a bowl and add carrot cheese and season with pepper
4. Toss well and split the mixture between the portions
5. Toss and enjoy!

(the dressing and salad should be in various containers)

Satisfying Spinach Dip

Serving: 4
Prep Time: 4 minutes
Cook Time: 0 minutes
Ingredients 10 oz Spinach, raw
1 and a 1/2 Greek yogrut
1 tablespoon of onion powder
1/2 a teaspoon of garlic salt
Black pepper to taste
1/2 a teaspoon of Greek Seasoning
How To
Combine listed ingredients in a blender Emulsify Season and serve
Nutrition (Per Serving)
Calories: 101
Fat: 4g
Net Carbohydrates: 4g
Protein: 10g
Storage Options/Meal Prep Tips: Store the portions in airtight containers in your refrigerator for approximately 2-3 days.

Satisfying Ginger Soup

Serving: 4
Prep Time: 9 minutes
Cook Time: 9 minutes
Ingredients

- 3 cups of green onions, diced
- 2 cups of mushrooms,
- sliced 3 tsp of fresh ginger,
- grated 3 tsp of garlic, minced
- 4 tbsp of keto favorable tamari
- 2 cups of bok choy, chopped
- 1 tablespoon of cilantro, chopped
- 3 tbsp of carrot, grated
- 1 can of each of diced tomatoes and peppers (or freshly prepared)
- 6 cups of vegetable broth

How To

1. bring the above-mentioned ingredients (except green onion) into a saucepan
2. Bring the mixture to a boil over medium-high heat
3. Reduce down warmth to cook and simmer for 6 minutes
4. Stir in green onions and carrots and cook for two minutes
5. Sprinkle cilantro and revel!

Store in refrigerator for 2-3 days and microwave before serving. Freezer-time 2-3 months.

Personal Veggie Pizza

Serving: 4

Prep Time: 5 min
Cook Time: 15 minutes
Ingredients
- 4 large Portobello mushroom caps
- 1 mediu vine tomato
- 4 oz fresh mozarella cheese
- 1/4 cup fresh basil, chopped
- 6 tbsp ofo reside oil
- 20 pepperoni pieces
- Salt and pepper as needed

How To
1. Prepare the mushroom and scrap out the internals, making sure to maintain only the shell
2. twist the cubes over and broil them
3. Coat the shell with 3 tbsp of olive oil and season with salt and pepper
4. Broil for 5 minutes longer
5. Slice the tomato to thin slices and put them on top of the mushroom
6. Garnish with fresh basil and add pepperoni, cubed cheese on top
7. Broil for 4 minutes longer to melt the cheese
8. Serve and enjoy!

Nutrition (Per Serving)
Calories: 227
Fat: 15g
Net Carbohydrates: 2g
Protein: 21g

Storage Options/Meal Prep Tips: Store the portions in airtight containers in your refrigerator for around 4-5 days.

Fancy Charred Garlic Artichokes

Serving: 6
Prep Time: 5 min
Cook Time: 30 minutes
Ingredients
- 2 large sized artichokes
- 1 quartered lemon
- 3/4 cup of olive oil
- 4 chopped up garlic cloves
- 1 teaspoon of salt
- 1/2 a teaspoon of ground black pepper

How To
1. Take a large sized bowl and add water
2. Squeeze lemon juice in the water
3. dip the top of the artichokes and cut them half-lengthwise
4. Bring the water to a boil and then add the artichokes, let them cook for 15 minutes
5. till they're being cooked, pre-heat your grill to medium-high
6. when the chokes are cooked, drain them and squeeze the remaining lemon wedges to a medium sized bowl
7. Stir in garlic and olive oil
8. Season with salt and pepper
9. Brush the chokes with the coat of garlic dip and set them on the skillet

10. Grill for 10 minutes, then makings sure to keep basting it from time to time
11. Serve the grilled artichokes with the remaining drops

Nutrition (Per Serving)
Calories: 237 Fat: 19g
Net Carbohydrates: 12g
Protein: 5g
Storage Options/Meal Prep Tips: Store the portions in airtight containers for approximately 2-3 days.

Healthy Cauliflower Curry

Serving: 6
Prep Time: 10 minutes
Cook Time: 45 minutes
Ingredients
- 1 cauliflower head
- 1 and a 1/2 cups of full fat yogurt
- 2 tbsp curry powder
- 1 teaspoon of paprika, smoke
- 1 tsp of pepper
- Juice of 1 lime
- 1 tsp salt 1/2 a teaspoon of black pepper
- 2 teaspoon of zest of lime Topping
- 1/4 cup sun dried tomatoes, drained
- 1/2 a cup of pine nuts
- 1 tablespoon of cilantro
- 2 tbsp of feta cheese, crumbled into balls
- 1/4 cup olive oil Clove of garlic

How To
1. Pre-heat your oven to 375-degree Fahrenheit

2. Take a baking sheet and line with parchment paper
3. Take a bowl and add the key ingredients (except cauliflower)
4. Rub the mixture all over the cauliflower head
5. Bake for 45 minutes until crispy
6. Let it cool
7. Insert garlic, sun dried tomatoes, half pine nuts into a blender and mix until thicken
8. Add the remaining ingredients (topping) and combine
9. Cut cauliflower heads into florets and move to shallow dish
10. Drizzle topping mix and serve
11. Enjoy!

(the cooked cauliflower and dressing should be in various containers)

Great Sautéed Zucchini

Serving: 6
Prep Time: 5 min
Cook Time: 30 minutes
Ingredients
- 1 tbsp of olive oil
- 1/2 a red onion, diced
- Salt and pepper as needed
- 4 zucchini, halved and chopped
- 1/2 a pound of fresh mushroom, sliced
- 1 tomato, diced
- 1 garlic clove, minced
- 1 teaspoon of Italian seasoning

How To
1. Take a large sized skillet and set it over medium heat
2. Add onion and Saute for two minutes
3. Season with some salt and pepper
4. Add zucchini into the skillet
5. when the zucchini is tender, add garlic and Italian seasoning along with the tomatoes
6. Cook well and enjoy!

Nutrition (Per Serving)
Calories: 230
Fat: 22g
Net Carbohydrates: 4g
Protein: 5g
Storage Options/Meal Prep Tips: Store the portions in airtight containers for about 2-3 days.

Fancy Charred Garlic Artichokes

Serving: 5
Prep Time: 5 min
Cook Time: 30 minutes
Ingredients
- 2 tbsp of coconut butter
- 1/2 a cup of roasted red pepper chopped
- 1 large sized finely chopped shallots
- 1 teaspoon of celery salt
- 1 tablespoon of seasoned salt
- 1 teaspoon of organic paprika
- 1 pinch of crushed red pepper flakes
- 4-5 cups of Cauliflower broken into florets
- 4 cup of vegetable broth

- Only a splash of apple cider vinegar
- 1 pinch fresh thyme
- 1 cup of organic coconut milk

How To
1. Take a heavy bottomed pot and add coconut oil over medium heat
2. Add chopped shallots and Saute for 3 minutes
3. Add chopped up and roasted pepper together with the seasonings
4. Stir well and cook for 2-3 minutes
5. Add cauliflower, fresh coriander and inventory Bring it to a simmer and cover the pot, cook for 5-10 minutes
6. Function in tiny batches and puree the soup with an immersion blender
7. Bring the entire blended soup back to your own pot and stir in coconut milk

Nutrition (Per Serving)
Calories: 221
Fat: 17g
Net Carbohydrates: 10g
Protein: 8g
Storage Options/Meal Prep Tips: Store the portions in airtight containers for about 2-3 days.

Cool Cucumber Soup

Serving: 4
Prep Time: 14 minutes
Cook Time: 0 min
Ingredients

- 2 tbsp of minced garlic
- 4 cups of English cucumbers, peeled and diced
- 1/2 a cup of onions, diced
- 1 tbsp of lemon juice
- 1 plus a 1/2 cups of vegetable broth
- 1/2 a teaspoon of salt
- 1 whole avocado, diced
- 1/4 tsp of fred pepper flakes
- 1/4 cup of diced parsley
- 1/2 a cup of Greek yogurt, plain

How To
1. bring the listed ingredients into a blender and emulsify by mixing them (except 1/2 a cup of sliced onions)
2. Blend until smooth
3. Pour into 4 servings and top with remaining cucumbers Enjoy!

Nutrition (Per Serving)
Calories: 169
Fat: 12g
Net Carbohydrates: 6g
Protein: 4g
Storage Options/Meal Prep Tips: Freeze the portions in individual containers with lids. Good for 2-3 months.

Extremely Healthy Guacamole

Serving: 6
Prep Time: 15 minutes
Cook Time: 0 minutes
Ingredients
- 3 large ripe avocados

- 1 large red onion, peeled and diced
- 4 tbsp of freshly squeeze lime juice
- Salt as needed
- Freshly ground black pepper as needed
- Cayenne pepper as needed

How To
1. Halve the avocados and discard the rock
2. Scoop the flesh out of 3 avocado halves and move to large glass jar
3. Mash well using fork
4. Add 2 tbsp of lime juice to mashed avocado and mix
5. Diced the rest of the avocado and add them into a different bowl
6. Add remaining juice and toss Combine diced avocado and mashed avocado
7. Add chopped onion and toss well Season with pepper, salt and cayenne pepper.

Nutrition (Per Serving)
Calories: 172
Fat: 15g
Net Carbohydrates: 11g
Protein: 2g
Storage Options/Meal Prep Tips: Store the portions in airtight containers for approximately 2-3 times and serve with carrot, celery or cucumber sticks. Freezer 2-3 months.

Crunchy Cauliflower Rice

Serving: 2
Prep Time: 5 min

Cook Time: 6 minutes

Ingredients
- 1 head of grated cauliflower head
- 1 tbsp of Soy Sauce
- 1 pinch of salt
- 1 pinch of black pepper
- 1 tbsp of Garlic Powder
- 1 tbsp of Sesame Oil

How To
1. Add cauliflower to a food processor and grate it
2. Take a pan and then add sesame oil, allow it to warm up over medium heat
3. Add grated cauliflower and pour soy sauce
4. Cook for 4-6 minutes
5. Season and enjoy!

Nutrition (Per Serving)
Calories: 329
Fat: 28g
Net Carbohydrates: 13g
Protein: 10g

Storage Options/Meal Prep Tips: Store the portions in airtight containers for about 2-3 days.

Amazing Spring Salad Serving: 1

Prep Time: 10-15 minutes

Cook Time: 0 minutes

- Ingredients 2 oz of Mixed Green Vegetables
- 3 tbsp of roasted pine nuts
- 2 tbsp of 5-minute 5 Keto Raspberry Vinaigrette
- 2 tbsp of Shaved Parmesan
- 2 slices of Bacon
- Salt as required

- Pepper as required

How To
1. Take a cooking pan and add bacon, cook the bacon until crispy
2. Take a bowl and add the salad ingredients and mix well, add crumbled bacon to the salad Mix well
3. Dress it with your favorite dressing

Nutrition (Per Serving)
Calories: 209
Fat: 17g
Net Carbohydrates: 10g
Protein: 4g

Chapter 12: Desert my favorite

Pumpkin and Cardamom Donuts

Serving: 4
Prep Time: 10 minutes
Cook Time: 22 minutes
Ingredients
- 3 whole large eggs
- 1 cup pumpkin puree
- 1/2 a cup of coconut flour
- 1/3 cup melted butter
- 2 tbsp of erythritol
- 1 teaspoon of Cardamom
- 2/4 tsp of liquid stevia
- 1/4 tsp vanilla extract
- 1/4 teaspoon of orange extract
- 1/4 tsp of salt

How To
1. Pre-heat your Oven to 325-degree Fahrenheit
2. Have a microwave proof bowl and add butter and microwave the butter
3. Fold in the wet ingredients and combine
4. Take another bowl and add the dry ingredients, mix well and transfer the dry ingredients into the wet ingredients and mix
5. Roll up the dough into balls and put them in a cupcake tray
6. Bake for 18-22 minutes until they are slightly browned

7. Once cooled, dust with cinnamon and simmer with a little bit of maple syrup.

Blueberry Morning Scones

Serving: 12
Prep Time: 10 minutes
Cook Time: 15 minutes
Ingredients
- 3 large eggs, beaten
- 1 plus a 1/2 cups of almond milk
- 3/4 cup of fresh/frozen raspberries
- 1/2 a cup of stevia
- 2 teaspoon of pure vanilla extract
- 2 tsp of baking powder

How To
1. Pre-heat your Oven to 375-degree Fahrenheit
2. Take a baking sheet and carefully line it with baking paper, keep the prepared sheet on the side
3. Take a large mixing bowl and add eggs, stevia, vanilla extract, baking powder and almond milk
4. Whisk the mixture well
5. Fold in raspberries and stir
6. Scoop the batter on your baking sheet and make mounds (keep 2 inch space between each mound)
7. Bake for 15 minutes and transfer to cooling rack
8. Let them cool for 10 minutes Enjoy!

Nutrition (Per Serving)
Calories: 133
Fat: 8g

Net Carbohydrates: 4g
Protein: 2g
Storage Options/Meal Prep Tips: Transfer the scones into an air tight container and store in a cool and dry location for 5 days. As an alternative, you can refrigerate them for up to 5 times. Be certain that you re-heat before serving!

Deliciously Chocolate Coated Bacon

Serving: 6
Prep Time: 15 minutes
Cook Time: 20 minutes
Ingredients
- 12 bacon slices
- 4 plus a 1/2 tbsp of unsweetened dark chocolate
- two and a 1/4 tbsp of coconut oil
- 1 plus a 1/2 teaspoon of liquid stevia

How To
1. Pre-heat your Oven to 425-degree Fahrenheit
2. Skewer bacon to iron skewers
3. Arrange the skewers on a baking sheet
4. Bake for 15 minutes until crispy Transfer to cooling rack
5. Take a saucepan and put it over low heat, add coconut oil and melt it simmer in chocolate and melt
6. Add stevia and stir Put crispy bacon onto a sheet of parchment paper and coat with chocolate mixture allow the chocolate dry and Solidify Enjoy!

Nutrition (Per Serving)
Calories: 258
Fat: 26g
Net Carbohydrates: 0.5g
Protein: 7g
Storage Options/Meal Prep Tips: Transfer to airtight containers and serve when necessary, potential to simmer for 5 days.

Easy Bake Coconut Macaroons

Serving: 18
Prep Time: 2 hours 20 minutes
Cook Time: 0 minutes
Ingredients
- 1 plus a 1/2 cups of shredded unsweetened coconut
- 3/4 cup of fullfat unsweetened coconut milk
- 2 plus a 1/4 teaspoon of stevia

How To
1. bring the listed ingredients into a bowl
2. Mix them well and tightly cover the mixture with plastic wrap
3. Refrigerate for two hours
4. After chilled, scoop the coconut mixture into chunks and serve!

Nutrition (Per Serving)
Calories: 47
Fat: 5g
Net Carbohydrates: 2g
Protein: 0.4g

Storage Options/Meal Prep Tips: Store the balls in airtight containers and serve when needed, may be kept in fridge for up to 3 times.

Raspberry Popsicles
Serving: 4
Prep Time: 120 minutes
Cook Time: 0 minutes
Ingredients
- 3 plus a 1/2 oz of Raspberries
- Juice of 1/2 a lemon
- 1/4 cup of coconut oil
- 1 cup of coconut milk
- 1/4 cup of sour cream
- 1/4 cup of thick cream
- 1/2 a teaspoon of Guar Gum
- 20 drops of Liquid Stevia

How To
1. Take an immersion blender and toss in all the ingredients and combine them completely nicely
2. Once done, take them mix through a net and strain the mixture, discarding all the raspberry seeds
3. Pour in the mixture into a mould and keep the mould in the refrigerator for 2 hours
4. After done, pass the mould through warm water to dislodge the popsicles

Nutrition (Per Serving)
Calories: 65
Fat: 1g

Net Carbohydrates: 8g
Protein: 3g

Secret Yogurt Parfait

Serving: 4
Prep Time: 10 minutes
Cook Time: 0 minutes
Ingredients
- 1 cup walnuts, toasted
- Sweetener like stevia (as needed)
- 1 cup shredded coconut
- 2 cups of total fat yogurt
- 4 couple blueberries
- 4 couple berries
- 4 bananas, sliced
- 1 cup toasted flax seeds
- 1 cup of Macadamia pieces

How To
1. Take a mason jar and add 3 tablespoons of yogurt into the underside
2. Add sweetener then make layers of nuts, carrots and coconut, making sure to keep switching between ingredients while creating the layers
3. Pour the rest of the yogurt on top Enjoy!

Nutrition (Per Serving)
Calories: 230
Fat: 15g
Net Carbohydrates: 9g
Protein: 20g

Choco Peanut Fat Bombs
Serving: 8
Prep Time: 75 minutes
Cook Time: 0 min
Ingredients
- 2 tbsp of butter
- 2 tbsp of coconut oil
- 2 tablespoon of heavy cream
- 1 tbsp of peanut butter
- 1 tbsp of unsweetened cocoa powder
- 1/2 a teaspoon of vanilla extract
- 1/2 a teaspoon of liquid stevia

How To
1. Add peanut butter, coconut oil, butter in a microwave proof bowl and microwave at 10 second intervals until completely melted
2. Stir the mixture and add heavy cream and blend
3. Add cocoa powder, vanilla extract and stevia and stir
4. Pour the mixture into ice cube tray with 8 chambers and freeze for 1 hour
5. Serve and enjoy!

Nutrition (Per Serving)
Calories: 73
Fat: 8g
Net Carbohydrates: 1g
Protein: 0.6g
Storage Options/Meal Prep Tips: Potential to chill for two weeks in refrigerator.

Creamy and Satisfying Vanilla Pudding

Serving: 4
Prep Time: 5 min
Cook Time: 12 minutes
Ingredients 2 large egg yolks
1 cup of 36% heavy cream
1 plus a 1/2 teaspoon of stevia
1 teaspoon of arrowroot flour
1/2 a teaspoon of pure vanilla extract
Sea salt as needed
How To
1. Take a heavy-duty saucepan and add egg yolk
2. Whisk in cream, stevia, arrowroot flour, pure vanilla extract and mix well
3. Season with salt and stir
4. Put it over moderate heat and stir until the mixture just starts to steam
5. Reduce heat to low and keep stirring for 10 minutes
6. Pour pudding into 4 heatproof containers
7. Serve and enjoy!

Nutrition (Per Serving)
Calories: 135
Fat: 13g
Net Carbohydrates: 2g
Protein: 2g
Storage Options/Meal Prep Tips: For keeping it, put a sheet of plastic wrap on top and refrigerate for up to 3 times

Conclusion

I can not say how honored I am to believe you found my book informative and interesting enough to read it all through to the finish. From here on out, I'd encourage you to continue experimenting with unique components and walk towards the path of becoming the next master of the arts of meal prep! I thank you for buying this book and I hope that you had as much fun reading it as I had writing it.

Printed in Great Britain
by Amazon